HERBAL REMEDIES FOR ECZEMA

Unlocking Nature's Healing Power With Herbs For Flourishing Skin, Holistic Wellness, Lasting Relief And Healthy Lifestyle

DR. CARDEN KYRIE

DISCLAIMER

The only goal of this book is informational. Every effort has been taken by the author and publisher to ensure that the information provided is accurate. But the material in this book is given "as is," without any express or implied representation, warranty, or condition as to its accuracy, completeness, or suitability for any particular purpose.

Any loss, damage, or injury resulting from using the information in this book, or from any action or decision made as a result of such use, will not be covered by the author's or publisher's liability. It is recommended that readers seek the assistance of a certified specialist for guidance specific to their situation.

The opinions and viewpoints conveyed in this book belong to the author and may not necessarily represent the official stance or policies of any specified organizations or people. Any likeness to real-life occurrences, places, or people—living or deceased—is wholly coincidental.

No specific product, service, or therapy discussed in this book is endorsed by the author or publisher. Any reference to goods or services is made only for informative reasons and is not intended as a recommendation or endorsement.

Before making any judgments or acting on any information, readers are urged to independently confirm it all. Any unfavorable effects or repercussions arising from the usage of the material included in this book are disclaimed by the author and publisher.

By using this book, you consent to absolving the publisher and author of any and all claims, obligations, or losses resulting from your use of the material in it.

I appreciate your cooperation and understanding.

TABLE OF CONTENTS

CHAPTER ONE

INTRODUCTION TO ECZEMA

COMPREHENDING PEDIATRIC ECZEMA

Eczema is a prevalent problem, particularly in children. Eczema is a persistent skin disorder marked by inflammation and irritation. Parents, caregivers, and medical professionals must comprehend pediatric eczema. Red, itchy rashes are a common symptom of this illness, which can cause the kid discomfort as well as worry. Examining the complexities of childhood eczema entails investigating its origins, manifestations, and possible initiators, offering an all-encompassing viewpoint on handling and reducing its influence on early life.

Recognizing the complexity of eczema in children is essential to understanding it. Eczema is frequently associated with a hereditary and environmental cocktail. Knowing that there is a genetic predisposition to eczema makes it possible to take preventative steps, such as early identification and management of potential triggers. Furthermore, stress, irritants, and allergens can all worsen the symptoms of eczema. Thus, developing successful techniques for managing and avoiding flare-ups of eczema requires a comprehensive understanding of a child's environment and genetic composition.

THE VALUE OF NATURAL TREATMENTS

The significance of natural therapies for eczema cannot be emphasized, even with the wide range of medications available. An alternate strategy that fits with the expanding movement toward holistic well-being is provided by natural medicines. These treatments frequently have an emphasis on mild, non-invasive techniques that try to nourish and calm the skin without having the possible negative consequences of some pharmaceutical therapies. Natural therapies are important because they can alleviate symptoms while lowering the possibility of negative reactions. This is particularly important in the sensitive setting of pediatric care.

As part of a larger trend toward a more conscientious and sustainable approach to healthcare, parents and caregivers are increasingly resorting to natural therapies. Adopting natural solutions for children's eczema entails investigating a variety of choices, such as herbal medications, essential oils, and dietary modifications. By taking this approach, caregivers aim to treat the underlying causes of eczema and enhance general skin health, creating a balance that benefits the child's overall health.

Comprehending childhood eczema necessitates a careful examination of all of its facets, from inherited tendencies to external stimulants. Among the many options for therapy, the importance of natural therapies stands out as a crucial factor. This move toward natural therapies highlights a more comprehensive strategy that puts the child's general health and well-being first, to reduce the negative effects of potentially harsh interventions while simultaneously symptomatic relief. When discussing eczema and how to treat it, individuals involved in the care and welfare of children with this skin condition need to have a comprehensive and knowledgeable viewpoint.

CHAPTER TWO

WHAT IS DERMATITIS?

ECZEMA: DEFINITION AND TYPES

Dermatitis, another name for eczema, is a persistent skin disorder marked by redness, itching, and inflammation. It is a word often used to characterize a class of skin conditions involving the immune system's reaction to certain allergens or irritants. Eczema is a group of illnesses that impact the outer layer of the skin rather than a single illness. Atopic dermatitis, contact dermatitis, dyshidrotic eczema, nummular eczema, and seborrheic dermatitis are the most prevalent kinds of eczema.

One of the most common types of eczema, atopic dermatitis typically manifests in early childhood or infancy. It has a hereditary basis and is frequently connected to other allergic reactions including hay fever and asthma. On the other hand, direct contact with allergens or irritants causes contact dermatitis, which is characterized by skin inflammation. Mostly affecting the hands and feet, dyshidrotic eczema is characterized by severe itching and blistering. Coin-shaped lesions on the skin are the hallmark of nummular eczema, whereas seborrheic dermatitis usually affects parts of the skin with a high concentration of oil glands, such as the face and scalp.

CHILDHOOD PREVALENCE

Eczema is a common skin disorder in children that frequently presents as atopic dermatitis. Although the precise origin of atopic dermatitis is unknown, a mix of environmental and genetic factors is thought to be involved. Children who have a family history of allergies may be at higher risk of getting eczema. Children's eczema prevalence has increased recently, possibly due to a combination of variables including environmental exposures, hygienic habits, and lifestyle changes.

TYPICAL TRIGGERS

The common causes of flare-ups of eczema differ from person to person. Exposure to certain allergies, irritants, or harsh weather conditions is examples of environmental factors that might aggravate symptoms. In certain people, specific foods—like dairy, eggs, almonds, and soy—can also cause eczema. Infections, hormonal fluctuations, and stress can all contribute to the onset or worsening of eczema symptoms. It's essential to comprehend and recognize these triggers to manage and stop flare-ups.

A variety of strategies are used to manage eczema, such as hydrating the skin, avoiding recognized irritants, taking prescription medicine, and making lifestyle adjustments. Emollients and topical corticosteroids are frequently administered as means of symptom relief and inflammation reduction. Immunosuppressive medicines or systemic treatments may be advised in extreme situations.

Working together with medical professionals to create a customized treatment plan that targets unique triggers and symptoms is crucial for people with eczema.

A collection of long-term skin disorders including inflammation, redness, and itching are together referred to as eczema. Gaining knowledge about the various forms of eczema, including seborrheic dermatitis, atopic dermatitis, contact dermatitis, dyshidrotic eczema, and nummular eczema, might help one appreciate how varied this ailment is. Atopic dermatitis is a common kind of eczema in children, and its development is influenced by both environmental and hereditary factors. Effectively controlling eczema and enhancing the quality of life for those afflicted with this condition requires identifying and addressing frequent triggers, which can range from environmental factors to stress and nutritional components.

CHAPTER THREE

CONVENTIONAL THERAPIES FOR PEDIATRIC ECZEMA

TRADITIONAL DRUGS

Conventional drugs are frequently used in traditional treatments for childhood eczema to control symptoms and offer relief. These drugs are intended to relieve the discomfort, itching, and inflammation brought on by eczema, a chronic skin disease marked by red, itchy rashes. Traditional drugs can play a crucial role in the overall management strategy, helping to reduce flare-ups and enhance the quality of life for kids with eczema.

TOPICAL STEROIDS

Topical steroids are one of the most often prescribed drug types for childhood eczema. These drugs, which are available in different potencies and combinations, function by lowering inflammation and inhibiting the immune system in the afflicted skin regions. Topical steroids are frequently used topically on the skin, focusing on the areas where eczema flare-ups occur. Even if they work well to relieve pain, long-term usage of these products may cause negative effects such as skin thinning, discoloration, and the formation of stretch marks.

ANTI-HISTAMINES

Another type of conventional drug that is frequently used to treat pediatric eczema is antihistamines. Histamine, a substance generated during allergic reactions that contributes to itching, is the main target of these drugs. Antihistamines, which block histamine receptors, can help children with eczema sleep better and feel less itchy. It's crucial to remember that although antihistamines can reduce itching, they might not immediately deal with the underlying inflammation that underlies eczema.

ANTIBODIES THAT SUPPRESS THE IMMUNE SYSTEM

Immunosuppressants may be taken into consideration in more severe cases of infantile eczema when alternative treatments have proven to be ineffective. By inhibiting the immune system, these drugs lessen inflammation, which in turn lessens the symptoms of eczema. Immunosuppressant has possible hazards and side effects, such as an increased susceptibility to infections, even if they can be useful in treating eczema. To weigh the advantages and potential hazards of immunosuppressant use in children, medical personnel must closely observe the patient.

CONSTRAINTS AND ADVERSE REACTIONS

Conventional drugs are useful in treating the symptoms of childhood eczema, but their use has significant drawbacks and possible adverse consequences. Extended application of topical steroids may cause skin thinning, and an excessive dependence on these drugs may conceal underlying problems. Antihistamines don't treat the underlying cause of eczema; they just relieve itching. Furthermore, despite their strength, immunosuppressant may be harmful to a child's general health because of how they affect the immune system.

Moreover, each child will react differently to these drugs, so what works for one child could not work as well for another. Healthcare providers must carefully assess each kid with eczema's unique needs, taking into account the child's age, the severity of the condition, and the possibility of adverse effects. Furthermore, a thorough strategy for managing eczema frequently entails a mix of prescription drugs, skincare regimens, and lifestyle modifications catered to the particular requirements of each child. To track the child's development and modify the treatment plan as needed, regular follow-up visits and communication between parents and healthcare professionals are crucial.

CHAPTER FOUR

THE BENEFITS OF NATURAL TREATMENTS ADVANTAGES OF NATURAL METHODS

Natural therapies emphasize long-term health and total well-being, providing a plethora of advantages that go beyond simple symptom relief. One of the main benefits is that these treatments are mild and non-invasive, and they frequently cause fewer side effects than synthetic drugs. Numerous natural therapies make use of the therapeutic qualities of plants, herbs, and other natural ingredients to address a range of health issues in a more harmonious and well-rounded manner.

The advantages of using natural therapies for healing go beyond the physical to include psychological and emotional benefits. The focus on holistic well-being acknowledges the complex relationship between the mind and body and the critical roles that mental and emotional wellness play in general wellness. Herbal medicine, aromatherapy, and mindfulness practices are examples of practices that not only treat physical ailments but also promote emotional equilibrium, mental clarity, and inner harmony.

CHILDREN'S HOLISTIC HEALING

Given the interdependence of mental, emotional, and physical health, holistic healing for kids is a crucial component of natural therapies. In contrast to many traditional therapies that might only target symptom relief, holistic methods take into account the full child. By addressing the underlying causes of health problems, this holistic approach fosters resilience and general well-being. Natural treatments for kids often include dietary changes, lifestyle modifications, and mild therapies that assist their growing bodies and brains without putting them in needless danger. Beyond treating particular conditions, holistic therapy for kids involves building a strong foundation for their long-term health. Natural child cures frequently center on preventive practices, such as eating a healthy diet, getting enough sleep, and practicing stress management. Holistic approaches help children develop long-term resilience by establishing good habits at a young age, giving them the skills they need to face obstacles in life while maintaining strong mental and physical health.

COMBINING CONVENTIONAL TREATMENTS WITH NATURAL REMEDIES

Combining conventional medical procedures with herbal remedies is a forward-thinking, all-encompassing approach to healthcare. This integration, which acknowledges the benefits of both conventional and alternative medicine, enables a more individualized and successful treatment approach. Natural therapies, for example, can assist the body's natural healing processes, boost immunity, and reduce side effects in addition to orthodox treatments. For those wanting a comprehensive approach to their well-being, this cooperative strategy creates a synergy that can maximize health results and increase overall quality of life.

The combination of conventional therapies and natural remedies recognizes the benefits of each strategy while addressing its drawbacks. This collaborative methodology is especially useful for complex or chronic health disorders, where a multimodal approach may provide better outcomes. Patients gain from the combined knowledge of conventional and natural medicine professionals, and they receive a thorough, personalized treatment plan that takes into account their particular requirements and preferences.

The argument in favor of natural medicines is based on the holistic advantages they provide, stressing the importance of an all-encompassing strategy for wellness. When these treatments are given to kids, they form an essential part of holistic rehabilitation, promoting their mental, emotional, and physical health.

CHAPTER FIVE

FINDING AND STEERING CLEAR OF TRIGGERS

TYPICAL ENVIRONMENTAL STRESSORS

One of the most important aspects of treating a variety of health disorders, especially those about allergies, sensitivities, and dietary concerns, is recognizing and avoiding triggers. Typical environmental triggers are a wide range of substances that have the potential to cause negative reactions in people. For example, allergens are compounds that can cause allergic reactions. These can include dust mites, pollen, animal dander, and specific compounds. For those who are more susceptible to allergic reactions, identifying and reducing exposure to certain allergens is crucial.

ANGRY PEOPLE

Analogously, irritants constitute an additional class of environmental triggers that have the potential to worsen pre-existing health conditions.

These irritants can include certain cleaning agents, smoking, pollution, and strong scents. Since each person is sensitive to these substances differently, it is critical to recognize these irritants and either minimize or completely avoid exposure to avoid negative reactions.

NUTRITIONAL STRESSORS

In managing one's health, dietary triggers are essential, especially for people with food allergies and sensitivities. Food allergies are characterized by a range of symptoms from minor discomfort to severe reactions caused by the immune system's reactivity to particular proteins in particular meals. People who have a history of food allergies should carefully read ingredient labels and be mindful of cross-contamination hazards.

Food elimination is another tactic used to recognize and control food triggers. These diets entail methodically cutting out particular foods or food groups from the diet for a predefined amount of time, then gradually reintroducing them to see if there are any negative effects. This technique can be used to identify the foods that may be causing health problems, which makes it useful for treating autoimmune illnesses or ailments like irritable bowel syndrome (IBS).

ALLERGIES TO FOOD

One group of dietary factors that can cause severe and potentially fatal reactions is food allergies. People who have been diagnosed with food allergies should strictly avoid all allergenic foods and carry an auto-injector of epinephrine in case of an emergency. Preventing unintentional contact with allergies is mostly dependent on education and awareness, especially in social or dining contexts.

Recognizing and avoiding triggers requires a thorough awareness of food components, environmental circumstances, and particular allergens. A proactive approach to managing environmental and dietary triggers, such as food allergies and elimination diets, or identifying and reducing exposure to common triggers in the environment, such as allergens and irritants, is crucial for people who want to keep their health and well-being.

CHAPTER SIX

REJUVENATION FROM WITHIN ECZEMA DIET RICH IN NUTRIENTS FOODS FOR HEALTHY SKIN

Chronic inflammatory skin conditions like eczema often require a multimodal approach to healing, with nutrition being a key component. Eating foods high in nutrients is a basic way to promote skin health from the inside out. Important elements that support skin health and renewal include zinc, vitamins A, C, and E. Nuts, bright fruits, and leafy green vegetables are excellent providers of these micronutrients. Furthermore, walnuts, flaxseeds, and salmon all include fatty acids that can help lower inflammation, which is important for controlling eczema symptoms.

Antioxidants found in vegetables like tomatoes and fruits like berries also aid in the fight against oxidative stress, which can worsen the symptoms of eczema. Eating a wide variety of nutrient-dense meals boosts general immune function and gives the body the building blocks it needs for skin regeneration, promoting a holistic approach to internal healing.

THE VALUE OF HYDRATION

The foundation of healthy skin is hydration, which is especially important for those with eczema. Drinking enough water keeps the skin supple, keeps it from drying up, and aids in the body's natural detoxifying processes. Dehydrated skin is more prone to irritation and inflammation, which can exacerbate the symptoms of eczema. As a result, adding enough water to one's daily regimen is an easy yet effective way to take care of one's skin from the inside out.

Herbal teas and meals high in water content, such as cucumber and watermelon, can help maintain optimal hydration levels in addition to water. It's also crucial to refrain from consuming large amounts of dehydrating liquids, including coffee or sugary drinks. People with eczema can lay the groundwork for healthy skin and possibly even reduce some of the discomfort that comes with the condition by drinking enough water.

PROBIOTICS AND SUPPLEMENTS

In the fight for healthy skin, supplements can be invaluable allies, particularly for those who suffer from eczema. Supplements containing omega-3 fatty acids, which come from algae or fish oil, have shown anti-inflammatory qualities that may help control eczema symptoms. Supplementing with vitamin D can also be helpful because vitamin D deficiency has been connected to several skin disorders, including eczema.

Furthermore, the gut-skin relationship emphasizes how important probiotics are for managing eczema. Fermented foods such as kefir, sauerkraut, and yogurt include probiotics that help maintain a healthy gut microbiome. In turn, a healthy gut flora might enhance immunological response and lower inflammation, which may lessen the likelihood of eczema flare-ups. Supplements and probiotics combined with a well-rounded diet can improve the body's internal ecology and create the best possible conditions for skin healing.

Internal healing is a dynamic process that calls for the careful inclusion of foods high in nutrients, giving proper hydration priority, and taking probiotics and supplements into account. People with eczema can empower themselves to address the underlying causes of their problem and promote long-term skin health by adopting a holistic approach to eating.

CHAPTER SEVEN

EXTERNAL THERAPIES FOR CALMING THE SKIN

ORGANIC MOISTURIZERS

Natural moisturizers are essential for calming the skin and preserving its hydrated levels. These natural sources of nourishing characteristics for the skin make them excellent substitutes for commercial moisturizers. Coconut oil is a well-liked option that is notable for its many uses. Coconut oil, which is high in fatty acids, works well as a moisturizer by creating a barrier that shields the skin from the elements, keeping it from drying out, and encouraging a smooth, youthful complexion.

SHEA BUTTER

Another natural moisturizer praised for its emollient qualities is shea butter. Made from the nuts found on the shea tree, this butter is rich in fatty acids and vitamins, which help explain why it has such remarkable moisturizing properties. Shea butter is well renowned for its ability to relieve dryness, lessen inflammation, and support the suppleness of the skin. Because of its natural ingredients which typically don't include harsh chemicals like those found in some commercial products it is excellent for people with sensitive skin.

RELAXING SOAKS & BATHS

Additional external therapies for calming the skin include relaxing baths and soaks. For instance, oatmeal baths have long been used as a treatment for sensitive and inflamed skin. Beta-glucans, which are found in oats, have anti-inflammatory qualities that reduce redness and irritation. Oatmeal, when ground finely and added to a warm bath, creates a calming, milky solution that helps soothe skin disorders including dermatitis and eczema.

BATHS WITH EPSOM SALTS

Baths with Epsom salts offer an alternative method of calming the skin. Epsom salt, which is primarily composed of magnesium sulfate, is well-known for its capacity to soothe muscles and lower inflammation. It can produce a healing bath when dissolved in warm water, which may help relieve irritated or hurting skin. This is why people who are coping with ailments like psoriasis or tight muscles often choose Epsom salt baths.

TOPICAL APPLICATION OF HERBAL INFUSIONS

Another type of external therapy for calming the skin is herbal infusions for topical application. Many herbs can provide comfort for numerous skin conditions when infused into oils or applied as compresses. For example, chamomile, which has a reputation for being relaxing, is frequently applied topically to relieve inflamed skin. Lavender is another herb that may be added to baths or oils to have a relaxing impact on the skin because of its antibacterial and anti-inflammatory qualities.

Natural moisturizers like shea butter and coconut oil, relaxing baths like oatmeal and Epsom salt baths, and topical herbal infusions can all be used in conjunction with one another to help with exterior skin-soothing therapies. These methods, which emphasize the hydration and relaxation of the skin using organic and tried-and-true treatments, provide an alternative to commercial solutions.

CHAPTER EIGHT

MIND-BODY LINK
ECZEMA AND STRESS

Numerous disciplines, including psychology, medicine, and holistic health, are very interested in and researching the complex interaction between the mind and body. A noteworthy feature of the mind-body connection is how stress affects physical health, especially since it's linked to ailments like eczema. Stress is a potential trigger for flare-ups of eczema, frequently resulting from emotional or psychological issues.

Stress hormones are released by the body in response to stress, which can worsen inflammatory processes and cause skin reactions in people who are prone to eczema. Thus, it becomes essential to comprehend and manage stress to treat skin health and mental well-being holistically.

CHILDREN'S RELAXATION METHODS

Investigating strategies to reduce stress is crucial when examining the effects of the mind on the body, particularly in susceptible groups such as children. Children-specific relaxation methods are essential for fostering both physical and mental health. Like adults, children can suffer stress and anxiety, so it's critical to give them coping mechanisms to support their overall growth. It has been demonstrated that methods like guided visualization, deep breathing exercises, and mindfulness can help kid's better handle stress and develop emotional resilience.

Through the integration of these techniques into their everyday routines, kids can acquire essential abilities to effectively handle obstacles and foster healthy mental-physical equilibrium.

THE VALUE OF A HELPFUL ENVIRONMENT

An individual's surroundings can have a big impact on their physical and emotional well-being. This is especially true when it comes to the mind-body link and how important a supportive environment is. In addition to the physical surroundings, a supportive environment also includes the social and emotional components that enhance an individual's overall quality of life. A supportive environment helps counteract the harmful impacts of stress when it comes to managing illnesses like eczema. In addition to promoting a sense of security and resilience, emotional support from friends, family, and the community can help reduce stress. Furthermore, a physically cozy and secure setting can promote relaxation, which is good for one's physical and mental well-being.

The mind-body connection emphasizes how closely linked mental and physical health are. Stress, a ubiquitous element of contemporary life, can impact ailments such as eczema, underscoring the significance of stress mitigation in comprehensive medical therapy. Teaching kids how to relax turns into a wise investment in their long-term well-being. Last but not least, the importance of a supportive environment cannot be emphasized because it is critical in forming the mind-body link and promoting resilience and general health.

CHAPTER NINE

MODIFICATIONS TO LIFESTYLE FOR ECZEMA MANAGEMENT

OPTIONS FOR CLOTHES AND FABRICS

For people with eczema, choosing the appropriate clothes and materials is essential because some materials might make skin irritation worse. Choosing supple, airy textiles like cotton helps reduce abrasion and promote skin respiration. Wool and other rough, scratchy materials should be avoided since they might irritate delicate skin and cause flare-ups of eczema.

It is better to wear loose-fitting clothing because tight clothing might irritate the skin and generate friction. Additionally, avoiding needless rubbing and lowering the risk of skin irritation can be achieved by selecting clothing with smooth seams.

ESTABLISHING A SKIN-FRIENDLY ENVIRONMENT AT HOME

Keeping your house skin-friendly is essential to good eczema management. Frequent dusting and cleaning can lessen irritants and allergens that can aggravate eczema symptoms. Choosing hypoallergenic, fragrance-free cleaning supplies can reduce your exposure to harsh chemicals. In arid areas or throughout the winter, using a humidifier keeps the skin hydrated and helps avoid the itching and dryness that come with eczema. Using gentle, fragrance-free soaps and moisturizers as part of a regular skincare regimen helps maintain a better skin barrier.

SUNSCREEN AND DERMATITIS

Using sunscreen is essential for managing eczema because exposure to the sun can aggravate symptoms and cause discomfort for those with sensitive skin. Applying a high-SPF broad-spectrum sunscreen daily helps protect the skin from UV radiation. Choosing hypoallergenic sunscreens or sunscreens made especially for sensitive skin will help to further lower the chance of irritation. Putting on sun protection gear, such as wide-brimmed hats and long sleeves, adds another layer of defense against the sun. It's wise to seek shade when outside and stay out of direct sunshine during peak hours to reduce flare-ups of sun-induced eczema. For those with eczema, including these sun protection techniques in daily activities is crucial to promoting skin health and preventing symptom exacerbation.

CHAPTER TEN

INCLUDING NATURAL THERAPIES IN EVERYDAY LIVING

FORMULATING A PERSONALIZED THERAPY PROGRAM

A comprehensive strategy that takes into account all facets of a person's health is necessary when incorporating natural therapies into daily living. Creating a customized treatment plan is a crucial part of this procedure. This strategy should take into account lifestyle choices, individual health objectives, and medical circumstances. It's critical to comprehend one's body and recognize the places that need care. When creating a strategy that is workable and long-lasting, consideration should be given to elements including dietary choices, exercise regimens, and stress levels.

Depending on the needs of the patient, a customized treatment plan may include the use of herbs, vitamins, and other natural therapies. For example, if someone wants to strengthen their immune system, they should concentrate on including herbs like elderberry or echinacea in their regimen. Furthermore, dietary modifications like consuming more nutrient-dense meals can be very beneficial to general health. Natural therapies are guaranteed to be not only efficient but also easily incorporated into daily life with this customized approach.

KEEPING AN EYE ON AND MODIFYING REMEDIES

A durable natural remedy regimen must include both monitoring and remedy adjustments. Frequent self-evaluation enables people to monitor the success of the treatments they have selected and make any required modifications. Throughout this process, it's important to monitor any changes in symptoms, energy, and general well-being. Someone who uses herbal teas or meditation, for instance, to relieve stress may need to evaluate whether these treatments are having the desired effect. Maintaining the treatment plan's relevance to changing health demands requires flexibility in its adaptation.

SEEKING EXPERT ADVICE

Getting expert advice before incorporating natural therapies into daily life is a wise move. Even while self-care is important, speaking with a trained herbalist or medical expert can offer advice specific to a person's health issues. Experts can provide advice on proper dosages, possible drug interactions, and if particular treatments are suited for particular health issues. With this cooperative approach, people may confidently explore the wide world of natural therapies, knowing that their decisions are well-informed and in line with their overall health objectives.

Incorporating natural therapies into daily life requires a deliberate and customized strategy. A complete framework for integrating natural remedies into one's lifestyle includes creating a customized treatment plan, keeping an eye on and modifying treatments, and getting expert advice. People may make use of the advantages of natural medicines in a way that improves general well-being by understanding the special requirements of their bodies, remaining aware of their signals, and consulting professionals.